CW00556190

Keto (

Recipes

For Beginners

The Ultimate Keto Chaffle
Cookbook With 40
Mouthwatering And Low Carb
Recipes On A Budget.

Dorothy F. Brown

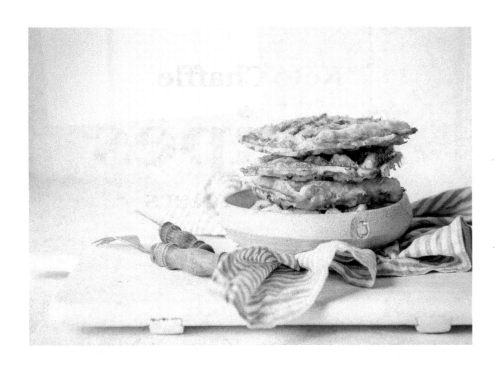

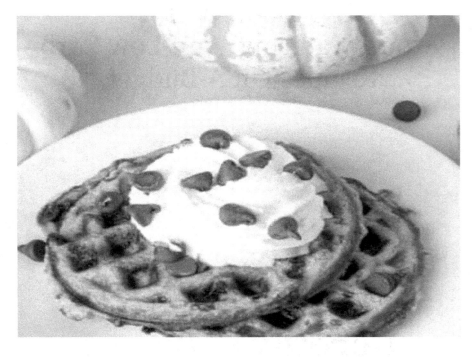

© **Copyright** 2021 by Dorothy F. Brown - All

rights reserved.

The following Book is reproduced below with the goal of providing information that is as accurate and reliable as possible. Regardless, purchasing this Book can be seen as consent to the fact that both the publisher and the author of this book are in no way experts on the topics discussed within and that any recommendations or suggestions that are made herein are for entertainment purposes only. Professionals should be consulted as needed prior to undertaking any of the action endorsed herein.

This declaration is deemed fair and valid by both the American Bar Association and the Committee of Publishers Association and is legally binding throughout the United States. Furthermore, the transmission, duplication, or reproduction of any of the following work including specific information will be considered an illegal act irrespective of if it is done electronically or in print. This extends to creating a secondary or tertiary copy of the work or a recorded copy and is only allowed with the express written consent from the Publisher. All additional right reserved.

The information in the following pages is broadly considered a truthful and accurate account of facts and as such, any inattention, use, or misuse of the information in question by the reader will render any resulting actions solely under their purview. There are no scenarios in which the publisher or the original author of this work can be in any fashion deemed liable for any hardship or damages that may befall them after undertaking information described herein.

Additionally, the information in the following pages is intended only for informational purposes and should thus be thought of as universal. As befitting its nature, it is presented without assurance regarding its prolonged validity or interim quality. Trademarks that are mentioned are done without written consent and can in no way be considered an endorsement from the trademark holder.

INTRODUCTION

Keto Diet is a high-fat, low-carb diet that is an increasingly popular way to lose weight. Keto is short for "ketosis", which occurs when the body has depleted its sugar stores, so it burns stored fat instead of glucose in order to produce energy.

Losing weight on a keto diet sounds pretty easy; just eat a few bacon sandwiches and you'll be slimmer in no time. However, there are drawbacks to this diet, including very low levels of vegetables and fruit (so important for fiber and other nutrients) as well as constipation from lack of dietary fiber. Here are some tips:

- It's important to drink plenty of water, not only because you may be eating more sodium than you need, but because staying hydrated will help your body process proteins and fats more efficiently.

- For best results, stay away from most fruits and vegetables. Some berries are allowed; others aren't. Vegetables that are considered "low in carbs" or "leafy greens" are fine—but there is a difference between low-carb and high-fiber. As a rule of thumb, if it looks like it has the texture of tree bark or is covered with seeds or bulbs (e.g., artichokes), it probably has a lot of carbs and should be avoided.

- Be careful with spices, which tend to have a lot of sugar; salt is OK. It can be easy to go overboard on spices.

- Eat plenty of salmon, tuna and egg whites. Meat—including beef, chicken, pork and lamb—should comprise 20 to 25 percent of your total diet. (Be aware that "lean" meat is often not very lean. Be prepared to trim off most of that fat before cooking.) A little bacon or sausage is fine, too.

- Avoid condiments and sauces, including barbecue sauce and ketchup. These are full of sugar and other unhealthy ingredients.

- Drink mostly water (or unsweetened drinks such as tea or coffee). Try to avoid drinks with a lot of added sugar, like fruit juice or alcohol. If you choose to drink wine, go for the dry stuff—red wine is best.

Now, for Chaffles.

What is Chaffle?

Keto chaffle recipe is a versatile and easy-to-make low carb pancake that only requires 2 ingredients. It's a way to satisfy your sweet cravings while staying keto!

Chaffle is made from cheese and eggs. You will need grated cheddar cheese (use any kind of cheese you have on hand) and eggs, beaten together, then fried in a pan with butter or coconut oil.

Chaffles are perfect for a low carb breakfast, lunch or dinner and can be a treat right out of the pan, with butter!

Why Keto and Chaffle is a perfect combination?

Keto Chaffle is a great way to satisfy your sweet cravings while staying 100% in ketosis. It helps you feel fuller for longer but at the same time it's not a high carb treat.

Chaffle gives you a lot of energy and it's an easy way to prepare breakfast if you want it to be ready quickly when you get up or even if you're in a hurry so it can be prepared on the go without any issues.

Keto Chaffle tastes amazing plain, with butter or with any toppings you like and it can also be used as sandwich bread substitute.

KETOGENIC DIET AND ITS BENEFITS

What is Ketogenic Diet?

The ketogenic diet is a low-carb, high-fat diet. This means that the macronutrient ratio of your diet should consist mainly of fat and protein with only a small percentage of carbohydrates.

The idea behind the ketogenic diet is to force your body to use fat rather than glucose as its primary fuel source. When we are in ketosis, we can function on almost any fuel source.

Benefits of the Ketogenic Diet

The benefits of the ketogenic diet are as follows:

1. No need to count calories.

On this diet, you can eat as much as you want. Since there are no grains, the carbohydrates in the diet are very low, and so you will not take in many calories.

2. There is no need to spend a lot of money on expensive foods.

Since this diet is high in fat, one of the cheapest sources of fat is chicken thighs and legs and other skinless poultry parts or meats from around the animal, such as organ meats (heart, liver, etc.).

3. Low levels of Beta-hydroxybutyrate (ketone body) is suitable for brain health

The ketogenic diet can increase the level of ketone bodies by 10 times than normal dietary levels through fat metabolism.

4. Decreased risk of heart disease

Many people can lower their LDL (bad) cholesterol by 75-90% and triglyceride levels by 60%.

5. Less inflammation

Because there are no carbohydrates in the ketogenic diet, your body becomes very efficient at burning ketones as fuel. This is excellent news if you have an autoimmune disorder like rheumatoid arthritis or Crohn's disease because inflammation is often linked to autoimmune problems.

6. Fast weight loss

People usually start losing weight within two weeks of starting the diet.

Volume (liquid)

US Customary	Metric
1/8 teaspoon	.6 ml
1/4 teaspoon	1.2 ml
1/2 teaspoon	2.5 ml
3/4 teaspoon	3.7 ml
1 teaspoon	5 ml
1 tablespoon	15 ml
2 tablespoon or 1 fluid ounce	30 ml
1/4 cup or 2 fluid ounces	59 ml
1/3 cup	79 ml
1/2 cup	118 ml
2/3 cup	158 ml
3/4 cup	177 ml
1 cup or 8 fluid ounces	237 ml
2 cups or 1 pint	473 ml
4 cups or 1 quart	946 ml
8 cups or 1/2 gallon	1.9 liters
1 gallon	3.8 liters

Weight (mass)

US contemporary (ounces)	Metric (grams)
1/2 ounce	14 grams
1 ounce	28 grams
3 ounces	85 grams
3.53 ounces	100 grams
4 ounces	113 grams
8 ounces	227 grams
12 ounces	340 grams
16 ounces or 1 pound	454 grams

Volume Equivalents (liquid)*

3 teaspoons	1 tablespoon	0.5 fluid ounce
2 tablespoons	1/8 cup	1 fluid ounce
4 tablespoons	1/4 cup	2 fluid ounces
5 1/3 tablespoons	1/3 cup	2.7 fluid ounces
8 tablespoons	1/2 cup	4 fluid ounces
12 tablespoons	3/4 cup	6 fluid ounces
16 tablespoons	1 cup	8 fluid ounces
2 cups	1 pint	16 fluid ounces

BASIC CHAFFLE RECIPES

1. Chaffle Sandwich With Bacon and Egg

Preparation time: 10 minutes

Cooking time: 5 minutes

Servings: 1

Ingredients

- 1 large egg
- 1/2 cup of shredded cheese
- thick-cut bacon
- fried egg
- sliced cheese

Directions

1. Preheat your waffle maker.
2. In a small mixing bowl, mix together egg and shredded cheese. Stir until well combined.
3. Pour one half of the waffle batter into the waffle maker. Cooking for 3-4 minutes or until golden brown. Repeat with the second half of the batter.
4. In a large pan over medium heat, cooking the bacon until crispy.
5. In the same skillet, in 1 tbsp. of reserved bacon drippings, fry the egg over medium heat. Cooking until desired doneness.
6. Assemble the sandwich, and enjoy!

Nutrition:

- Net Carbs: 5.7 g
- Calories: 358.8
- Total Fat: 25.1 g
- Saturated Fat: 4.3 g
- Protein: 26 g
- Carbs: 7.2 g
- Fiber: 1.5 g
- Sugar: 3.6 g

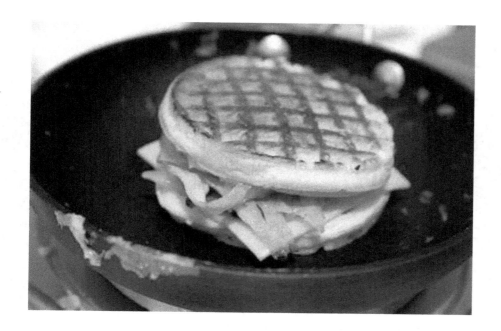

2. Bacon & Cheddar Cheese Chaffles

Preparation time: 5 minutes

Cooking time: 5 minutes

Servings: 6

Ingredients:

- ½ cup almond flour
- 3 bacon strips
- ¼ cup sour cream
- 1 ½ cup cheddar cheese
- ½ cup smoked Gouda cheese
- ½ tsp. onion powder
- ½ tsp. baking powder
- ¼ cup oat
- 1 egg
- 1 tbsp. oil
- 1 ½ tbsp. butter
- ¼ tsp. salt
- ½ tsp. parsley
- ¼ tsp. baking soda

Directions:

1. Heat the waffle maker.
2. Take a bowl add almond flour, baking powder, baking soda, onion powder, garlic salt and mix well.
3. In another bowl whisk eggs, bacon, cream, parsley, butter and cheese until well combined.
4. Now pour the mixture over dry ingredients and mix well.
5. Pour the batter over the preheated waffle maker and cooking for 5 to 6 minutes or until golden brown.
6. Serve the hot and crispy chaffles.

Nutrition:

- Net Carbs: 1.2 g
- Calories: 233.6
- Total Fat: 11.7 g
- Saturated Fat: 1.3 g
- Protein: 30.9 g
- Carbs: 1.2 g
- Fiber: 0g
- Sugar: 0 g

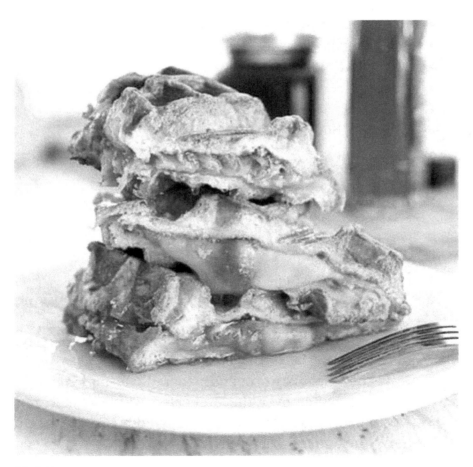

3. Jalapeno & Bacon Chaffle

Preparation time: 5 minutes

Cooking time: 5 minutes

Servings: 6

Ingredients:

- 3 tbsp. coconut flour
- 1 tsp. baking powder
- 3 eggs
- 8 oz. cream cheese
- ¼ tsp. salt
- 4 bacon slices
- 2 to 3 jalapenos
- 1 cup cheddar cheese

Directions:

1. Wash the jalapeno and slice them.
2. Take a pan and cooking jalapeno until golden brown or crispy.
3. Take a bowl add flour, baking powder and salt and mix.
4. In a mixing bowl add cream and beat well until fluffy.
5. Now in another bowl add egg and whisk them well.
6. Pour cream, cheese and beat until well combined.
7. Add the mixture with dry ingredients and make a smooth batter. After that fold the jalapeno in mixture.
8. Heat the waffle maker and pour the batter into it.
9. Cooking it for 5 minutes or until golden brown.
10. Top it with cheese, jalapeno and crème and serve the hot chaffles.

Nutrition:

- Net Carbs: 2.8 g
- Calories: 310
- Total Fat: 20 g
- Saturated Fat: 4.8 g
- Protein: 30.2 g
- Carbs: 3.1 g
- Fiber: 0.3 g
- Sugar: 1.2 g

4. Light & Crispy Bagel Chaffle Chips

Preparation time: 5 minutes

Cooking time: 5 minutes

Servings: 4

Ingredients:

- 3 tbsp. parmesan cheese
- 1 tsp. oil for grease
- 1 tsp. bagel seasoning
- Salt and pepper to taste

Directions:

1. Preheat the waffle maker.
2. Add the parmesan cheese in the pan and melt it well.
3. Now pour the melted parmesan cheese over the waffle maker and sprinkle bagel seasoning over the cheese.
4. Cooking the mixture for about 2 to 3 minutes without closing the lid.
5. Let it settle or turn crispy for 2 minutes then remove and serve the crispy chis crunch.

Nutrition:

- Net Carbs: 1.2 g
- Calories: 201.2
- Total Fat: 12.9 g
- Saturated Fat: 9.1 g
- Protein: 19.6 g
- Carbs: 1.5 g
- Fiber: 0.3 g
- Sugar: 0.7 g

5. Coconut Flour Waffle

Preparation time: 5 minutes

Cooking time: 5 minutes

Servings: 4

Ingredients

- 8 eggs
- 1/2 cup of butter or coconut oil (melted)
- 1 tsp. of vanilla extract
- 1/2 tsp. salt
- 1/2 cup of coconut flour

Directions:

1. Pre heat the mini waffle maker,
2. Whisk the eggs in a bowl,
3. Then you add the melted butter or coconut oil, cinnamon, vanilla and salt, mix properly then you add the Coconut flour.
4. Ensure the batter is thick,
5. Add the mixture into the mini waffle maker and allow to cooking till it has a light brown appearance.
6. Serve with butter or maple syrup.

Nutrition:

- Net Carbs: 6.8 g
- Calories: 357
- Total Fat: 28.9 g
- Saturated Fat: 13.2 g
- Protein: 15.2 g
- Carbs: 8.9 g
- Fiber: 2.1 g
- Sugar: 3.9 g

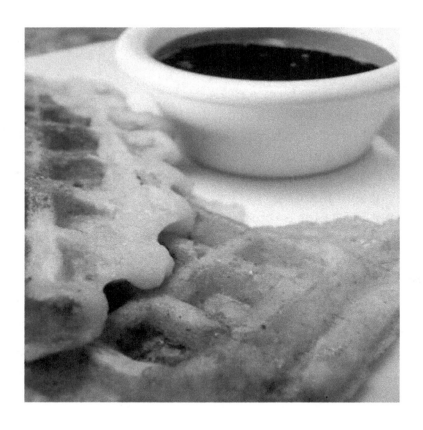

6. Cream Cheese Waffle

Preparation time: 10 minutes

Cooking time: 5 minutes

Servings: 4

Ingredients

- 2 cups of flour
- 1 tsp. baking powder
- 1/8 tsp. salt
- 2 tsp. light brown sugar
- 4 ounces of 1/3 Less Fat Cream Cheese,
- 2 eggs
- 1/2 cups of milk
- 2 tablespoons canola oil
- 1/2 tablespoon pure vanilla extract
- 4 tablespoons honey

Directions

1. First step is to preheat the mini waffle maker.
2. Then you mix the flour, baking powder, salt and light brown sugar; mix thoroughly to ensure uniformity.
3. In your bowl, add the cream cheese and egg yolks; mix until smooth.
4. Then you Add milk, oil and vanilla; mix properly.
5. Add flour mixture to cream cheese mixture and stir until moist. Set
6. The next step is to Place egg whites in a bowl and beat until it forms a stiff peak.
7. Using a spatula, fold the egg whites gently into the waffle-batter; fold just until thoroughly combined.

8. Pour 1/3-cup of the batter onto the preheated mini waffle iron.
9. Allow to cooking for about 2 to 3 minutes, or until it has a light brown appearance
10. Next step is to the Whipped Cream. Pour the heavy cream into a large mixing bowl and beat on until it becomes thick.
11. Add honey and continue to beat until soft peaks form. When ready,
12. Serve waffles topped with Honey Whipped Cream and fresh berries (if you prefer).

Nutrition:

- Net Carbs: 3.5 g
- Calories: 202.5
- Total Fat: 24.2 g
- Saturated Fat: 6 g
- Protein: 22.7 g
- Carbs: 4 g
- Fiber: 0.5 g
- Sugar: 1.1 g

7. Brownie Chaffle

Preparation time: 5 minutes

Cooking time: 3 minutes

Servings: 2

Ingredients

- 1 Egg Whisked
- 1/3 cup Mozzarella cheese Shredded
- 1 ½ tbsp. Cocoa Powder Dutch Processed
- 1 tbsp. Almond Flour
- 1 tbsp. Monkfruit Sweetener
- 1/4 tsp. Vanilla extract
- 1/4 tsp. Baking Powder
- Pinch of Salt
- 2 tsp. Heavy Cream

Directions

1. First step as always is to preheat your mini waffle iron.
2. Next, whisk the egg. Add the dry ingredients. Then add the cheese in a bowl. Then you Pour 1/3 of the batter on the waffle iron. Allow to cooking for 3 minutes or until steam stops coming out of the waffle iron.
3. Serve with your favorite low carb toppings.

Nutrition:

- Calories: 273
- Fat: 8.4 g
- Saturated Fat: 2.3 g
- Carbohydrate: 16.7 g
- Dietary Fiber: 2.2 g
- Protein: 30.7 g
- Cholesterol: 78 mg
- Sugars: 3.5 g
- Sodium: 1501 mg
- Potassium: 633 mg

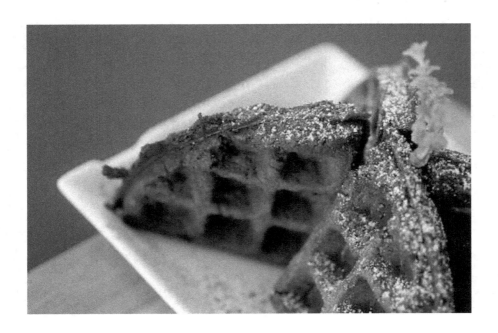

8. White Bread Keto Chaffle

Preparation time: 5 minutes

Cooking time: 4 minutes

Servings: 2

Ingredients

- 2 egg whites
- cream cheese, melted
- 2 tsp. water
- 1/4 tsp. baking powder
- 1/4 cup almond flour
- 1 Pinch of salt

Directions

1. Pre-heat the mini waffle maker,
2. Whisk the egg whites together with the cream cheese and water in a bowl.
3. Next step is to add the baking powder, almond flour and salt and whisk until you have a smooth batter. Then you pour half of the batter into the mini waffle maker.
4. Allow to cooking for roughly 4 minutes or until you no longer see steam coming from the waffle maker.
5. Remove and allow to cool.

Nutrition:

- Calories: 493
- Fat: 7.9 g
- Saturated Fat: 2 g
- Carbohydrate: 66.8 g
- Dietary Fiber: 14.2 g
- Protein: 40.1 g
- Cholesterol: 67 mg
- Sugars: 4.6 g
- Sodium: 88 mg
- Potassium: 1411 mg

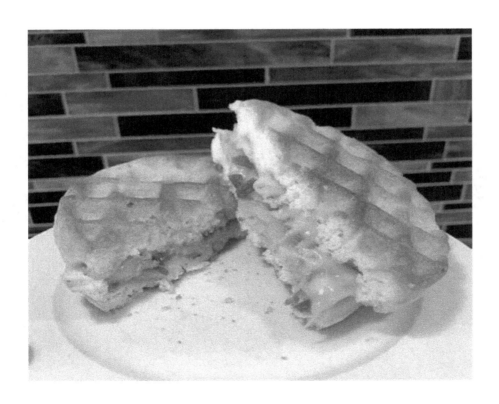

9. Pork Tzatziki Chaffle

Preparation time: 10 minutes

Cooking Time: 25 Minutes

Servings: 2

Ingredients:

- 4 eggs
- 2 cups grated provolone cheese
- Salt and pepper to taste
- 1 teaspoon dried rosemary
- 1 teaspoon dried oregano
- Pork loin
- 2 tablespoons olive oil
- 1 pound pork tenderloin
- Salt and pepper to taste
- Tzatziki sauce
- 1 cup sour cream
- Salt and pepper to taste
- 1 cucumber, peeled and diced
- 1 teaspoon garlic powder
- 1 teaspoon dried dill
- Other
- 2 tablespoons butter to brush the waffle maker

Directions:

1. Preheat the waffle maker.
2. Add the eggs, grated provolone cheese, dried rosemary, and dried oregano to a bowl. Season with salt and pepper to taste.
3. Mix until combined.
4. Brush the heated waffle maker with butter and add a few tablespoons of the batter.
5. Close the lid and cook for about 7 minutes depending on your waffle maker.
6. Meanwhile, heat the olive oil in a nonstick frying pan. Generously season the pork tenderloin with salt and pepper and cook it for about 7 minutes on each side.
7. Mix the sour cream, salt and pepper, diced cucumber, garlic powder and dried dill in a bowl.
8. Serve each chaffle with a few tablespoons of tzatziki sauce and slices of pork tenderloin.

Nutrition:

- Calories: 293
- Protein: 45 g
- Carbohydrates: 24 g
- Fats: 15 g

10. Mediterranean Lamb Kebabs on Chaffles

Preparation time: 10 minutes

Cooking Time: 15 Minutes

Servings: 2

Ingredients:

- 4 eggs
- 2 cups grated mozzarella cheese
- Salt and pepper to taste
- 1 teaspoon garlic powder
- ¼ cup Greek yogurt
- ½ cup coconut flour
- 2 teaspoons baking powder
- Lamb kebabs
- 1 pound ground lamb meat
- Salt and pepper to taste
- 1 egg
- 2 tablespoons almond flour
- 1 spring onion, finely chopped
- ½ teaspoon dried garlic
- 2 tablespoons olive oil
- Other
- 2 tablespoons butter to brush the waffle maker
- ¼ cup sour cream for serving
- 4 sprigs of fresh dill for garnish

Directions:

1. Preheat the waffle maker.
2. Add the eggs, mozzarella cheese, salt and pepper, garlic powder, Greek yogurt, coconut flour and baking powder to a bowl.
3. Mix until combined.
4. Brush the heated waffle maker with butter and add a few tablespoons of the batter.
5. Close the lid and cook for about 7 minutes depending on your waffle maker.
6. Meanwhile, add the ground lamb, salt and pepper, egg, almond flour, chopped spring onion, and dried garlic to a bowl. Mix and form medium-sized kebabs.
7. Impale each kebab on a skewer. Heat the olive oil in a frying pan.
8. Cook the lamb kebabs for about 3 minutes on each side.
9. Serve each chaffle with a tablespoon of sour cream and one or two lamb kebabs. Decorate with fresh dill.

Nutrition:

- Calories: 86
- Protein: 1.6 g
- Carbohydrates: 20 g
- Fats: 0.1 g

11. Creamy Bacon Salad on A Chaffle

Preparation time: 10 minutes

Cooking Time: 15 Minutes

Servings: 2

Ingredients:

- 4 eggs
- 1½ cups grated mozzarella cheese
- ½ cup parmesan cheese
- Salt and pepper to taste
- 1 teaspoon dried oregano
- ¼ cup almond flour
- 2 teaspoons baking powder
- Bacon salad
- ½ pound cooked bacon
- 1 cup cream cheese
- 1 teaspoon dried oregano
- 1 teaspoon dried basil
- 1 teaspoon dried rosemary
- 2 tablespoons lemon juice
- Other
- 2 tablespoons butter to brush the waffle maker
- 2 spring onions, finely chopped, for serving

Directions:

1. Preheat the waffle maker.
2. Add the eggs, mozzarella cheese, parmesan cheese, salt and pepper, dried oregano, almond flour and baking powder to a bowl.
3. Mix until combined.

4. Brush the heated waffle maker with butter and add a few tablespoons of the batter.
5. Close the lid and cook for about 7 minutes depending on your waffle maker.
6. Meanwhile, chop the cooked bacon into smaller pieces and place them in a bowl with the cream cheese. Season with dried oregano, dried basil, dried rosemary and lemon juice.
7. Mix until combined and spread each chaffle with the creamy bacon salad.
8. To serve, sprinkle some freshly chopped spring onion on top.

Nutrition:
- Calories: 336
- Protein: 34 g
- Carbohydrates: 8.29 g
- Fats: 13 g

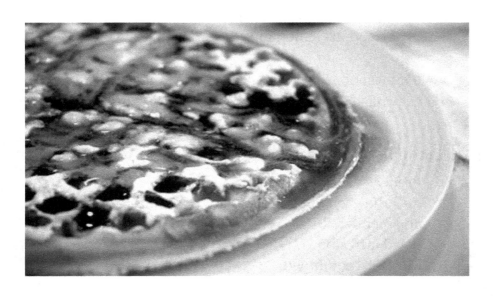

12. Beef & Sour Cream Chaffle

Preparation time: 10 minutes

Cooking Time: 15 Minutes

Servings: 2

- **Ingredients:**
- Batter
- 4 eggs
- 2 cups grated mozzarella cheese
- 3 tablespoons coconut flour
- 3 tablespoons almond flour
- 2 teaspoons baking powder
- Salt and pepper to taste
- 1 tablespoon freshly chopped parsley
- Seasoned beef
- 1 pound beef tenderloin
- Salt and pepper to taste
- 2 tablespoons olive oil
- 1 tablespoon Dijon mustard
- Other
- 2 tablespoons olive oil to brush the waffle maker
- ¼ cup sour cream for garnish
- 2 tablespoons freshly chopped spring onion for garnish

Directions:

1. Preheat the waffle maker.
2. Add the eggs, grated mozzarella cheese, coconut flour, almond flour, baking powder, salt and pepper and freshly chopped parsley to a bowl.
3. Mix until just combined and batter forms.

4. Brush the heated waffle maker with olive oil and add a few tablespoons of the batter.
5. Close the lid and cook for about 7 minutes depending on your waffle maker.
6. Meanwhile, heat the olive oil in a nonstick pan over medium heat.
7. Season the beef tenderloin with salt and pepper and spread the whole piece of beef tenderloin with Dijon mustard.
8. Cook on each side for about 4–5 minutes.
9. Serve each chaffle with sour cream and slices of the cooked beef tenderloin.
10. Garnish with freshly chopped spring onion.
11. Serve and enjoy.

Nutrition:

- Calories: 155
- Protein: 34 g
- Carbohydrates: 28 g
- Fats: 10 g

13. Pork Loin Chaffles Sandwich

Preparation time: 10 minutes

Cooking Time: 15 Minutes

Servings: 2

Ingredients:

- 4 eggs
- 1 cup grated mozzarella cheese
- 1 cup grated parmesan cheese
- Salt and pepper to taste
- 2 tablespoons cream cheese
- 6 tablespoons coconut flour
- 2 teaspoons baking powder
- Pork loin
- 2 tablespoons olive oil
- 1 pound pork loin
- Salt and pepper to taste
- 2 cloves garlic, minced
- 1 tablespoon freshly chopped thyme
- Other
- 2 tablespoons cooking spray to brush the waffle maker
- 4 lettuce leaves for serving
- 4 slices of tomato for serving
- ¼ cup sugar-free mayonnaise for serving

Directions:

1. Preheat the waffle maker.
2. Add the eggs, mozzarella cheese, parmesan cheese, salt and pepper, cream cheese, coconut flour and baking powder to a bowl.
3. Mix until combined.

4. Brush the heated waffle maker with cooking spray and add a few tablespoons of the batter.
5. Close the lid and cook for about 7 minutes depending on your waffle maker.
6. Meanwhile, heat the olive oil in a nonstick frying pan and season the pork loin with salt and pepper, minced garlic and freshly chopped thyme.
7. Cook the pork loin for about 5–minutes on each side.
8. Cut each chaffle in half and add some mayonnaise, lettuce leaf, tomato slice and sliced pork loin on one half.
9. Cover the sandwich with the other chaffle half and serve.

Nutrition:

- Calories: 436
- Protein: 4.7 g
- Carbohydrates: 50 g
- Fats: 24 g

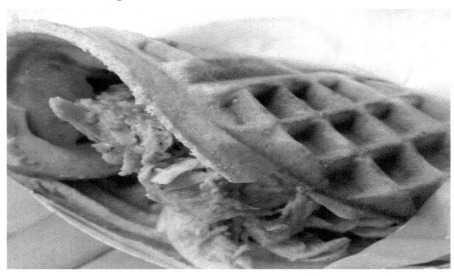

14. Beef Chaffles Tower

Preparation time: 10 minutes

Cooking Time: 15 Minutes

Servings: 2

Ingredients:

- Batter
- 4 eggs
- 2 cups grated mozzarella cheese
- Salt and pepper to taste
- 2 tablespoons almond flour
- 1 teaspoon Italian seasoning
- Beef
- 2 tablespoons butter
- 1 pound beef tenderloin
- Salt and pepper to taste
- 1 teaspoon chili flakes
- Other
- 2 tablespoons cooking spray to brush the waffle maker

Directions:

1. Preheat the waffle maker.
2. Add the eggs, grated mozzarella cheese, salt and pepper, almond flour and Italian seasoning to a bowl.
3. Mix until everything is fully combined.
4. Brush the heated waffle maker with cooking spray and add a few tablespoons of the batter.
5. Close the lid and cook for about 7 minutes depending on your waffle maker.

6. Meanwhile, heat the butter in a nonstick frying pan and season the beef tenderloin with salt and pepper and chili flakes.
7. Cook the beef tenderloin for about 5–minutes on each side.
8. When serving, assemble the chaffle tower by placing one chaffle on a plate, a layer of diced beef tenderloin, another chaffle, another layer of beef, and so on until you finish with the chaffles and beef.
9. Serve and enjoy.

Nutrition:

- Calories: 402
- Protein: 6 g
- Carbohydrates: 90 g
- Fats: 0.5 g

15. Turkey BBQ Sauce Chaffle

Preparation time: 10 minutes

Cooking Time: 8–10 Minutes

Servings: 2

Ingredients:

- Batter
- ½ pound ground turkey meat
- 3 eggs
- 1 cup grated Swiss cheese
- ¼ cup cream cheese
- ¼ cup BBQ sauce
- 1 teaspoon dried oregano
- Salt and pepper to taste
- 2 cloves garlic, minced
- Other
- 2 tablespoons butter to brush the waffle maker
- ¼ cup BBQ sauce for serving
- 2 tablespoons freshly chopped parsley for garnish

Directions:

1. Preheat the waffle maker.
2. Add the ground turkey, eggs, grated Swiss cheese, cream cheese, BBQ sauce, dried oregano, salt and pepper, and minced garlic to a bowl.
3. Mix everything until combined and batter forms.
4. Brush the heated waffle maker with butter and add a few tablespoons of the batter.
5. Close the lid and cook for about 8–10 minutes depending on your waffle maker.

6. Serve each chaffle with a tablespoon of BBQ sauce and a sprinkle of freshly chopped parsley.

Nutrition:

- Calories: 130
- Fat: 9.1 g
- Carbs: 12.1 g
- Protein: 1.3 g

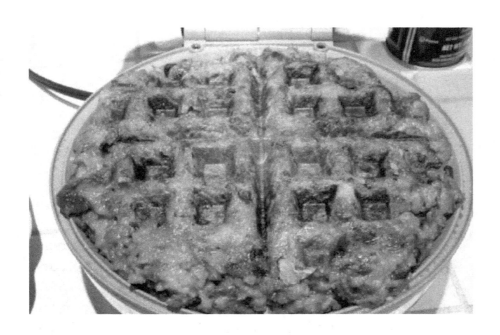

SAVORY CHAFFLE RECIPES

16. Italian Chicken and Basil Chaffle

Preparation time: 10 minutes

Cooking Time: 10 Minutes

Servings: 2

Ingredients:

- ½ pound ground chicken
- 4 eggs
- 3 tablespoons tomato sauce
- Salt and pepper to taste
- 1 cup grated Mozzarella cheese
- 1 teaspoon dried oregano
- 3 tablespoons freshly chopped basil leaves ½ teaspoon dried garlic
- 2 tablespoons butter to brush the waffle maker ¼ cup tomato sauce for serving
- 1 tablespoon freshly chopped basil for serving

Directions:

1. Preheat the waffle maker.
2. Add the ground chicken, eggs and tomato sauce to a bowl and season with salt and pepper.
3. Add the Mozzarella cheese and season with dried oregano, freshly chopped basil and dried garlic.
4. Mix until fully combined and batter forms.
5. Brush the heated waffle maker with butter and add a few tablespoons of the chaffle batter.

6. Close the lid and cooking for about 7-9 minutes depending on your waffle maker.
7. Repeat with the rest of the batter.
8. Serve with tomato sauce and freshly chopped basil on top.

Nutrition:

- Calories: 219
- Fat: 8 g
- Fiber: 4 g
- Carbs: 8 g
- Protein: 17 g

17. Beef Meatballs on A Chaffle

Preparation time: 10 minutes

Cooking Time: 20 Minutes

Servings: 4

Ingredients:

- Batter
- 4 eggs
- 2½ cups grated gouda cheese ¼ cup heavy cream
- Salt and pepper to taste
- 1 spring onion, finely chopped Beef meatballs
- 1 pound ground beef
- Salt and pepper to taste
- 2 teaspoons Dijon mustard
- 1 spring onion, finely chopped
- 5 tablespoons almond flour
- 2 tablespoons butter
- 2 tablespoons cooking spray to brush the waffle maker
- 2 tablespoons freshly chopped parsley

Directions:

1. Preheat the waffle maker.
2. Add the eggs, grated gouda cheese, heavy cream, salt and pepper and finely chopped spring onion to a bowl.
3. Mix until combined and batter forms.
4. Brush the heated waffle maker with cooking spray and add a few tablespoons of the batter.
5. Close the lid and cooking for about 7 minutes depending on your waffle maker.
6. Meanwhile, mix the ground beef meat, salt and pepper, Dijon mustard, chopped spring onion and

7. almond flour in a large bowl.
8. Form small meatballs with your hands.
9. Heat the butter in a nonstick frying pan and cooking the beef meatballs for about 3-4 minutes on each side.
10. Serve each chaffle with a couple of meatballs and some freshly chopped parsley on top.

Nutrition:

- Calories: 200
- Fat: 2 g
- Fiber: 3 g
- Carbs: 7 g
- Protein: 5 g

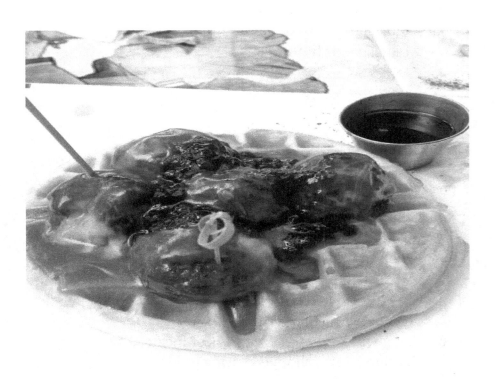

18. Mediterranean Lamb Kebabs on Chaffle

Preparation time: 10 minutes

Cooking Time: 15 Minutes

Servings: 4

Ingredients:

- 4 eggs
- 2 cups grated Mozzarella cheese Salt and pepper to taste
- 1 teaspoon garlic powder
- ¼ cup Greek yogurt
- ½ cup coconut flour
- 2 teaspoons baking powder Lamb kebabs
- 1 pound ground lamb meat
- Salt and pepper to taste
- 1 egg
- 2 tablespoons almond flour
- 1 spring onion, finely chopped ½ teaspoon dried garlic
- 2 tablespoons olive oil
- 2 tablespoons butter to brush the waffle maker ¼ cup sour cream for serving
- 4 sprigs of fresh dill for garnish

Directions:

1. Preheat the waffle maker.
2. Add the eggs, Mozzarella cheese, salt and pepper, garlic powder, Greek yogurt, coconut flour and baking powder to a bowl.
3. Mix until combined.
4. Brush the heated waffle maker with butter and add a few tablespoons of the batter.

5. Close the lid and cooking for about 7 minutes depending on your waffle maker.
6. Meanwhile, add the ground lamb, salt and pepper, egg, almond flour, chopped spring onion, and dried garlic to a bowl. Mix and form medium-sized kebabs.
7. Impale each kebab on a skewer. Heat the olive oil in a frying pan.
8. Cooking the lamb kebabs for about 3 minutes on each side.
9. Serve each chaffle with a tablespoon of sour cream and one or two lamb kebabs. Decorate with fresh dill.

Nutrition:

- Calories: 162
- Fat: 4 g
- Fiber: 5 g
- Carbs: 8 g
- Protein: 4 g

19. Beef and Sour Cream Chaffle

Preparation time: 10 minutes

Cooking Time: 15 Minutes

Servings: 4

Ingredients:

- Batter
- 4 eggs
- 2 cups grated Mozzarella cheese
- 3 tablespoons coconut flour
- 3 tablespoons almond flour
- 2 teaspoons baking powder
- Salt and pepper to taste
- 1 tablespoon freshly chopped parsley Seasoned beef
- 1 pound beef tenderloin
- Salt and pepper to taste
- 2 tablespoons olive oil
- 1 tablespoon Dijon mustard
- 2 tablespoons olive oil to brush the waffle maker ¼ cup sour cream for garnish
- 2 tablespoons freshly chopped spring onion for garnish

Directions:

1. Preheat the waffle maker.
2. Add the eggs, grated Mozzarella cheese, coconut flour, almond flour, baking powder, salt and pepper and freshly chopped parsley to a bowl.
3. Mix until just combined and batter forms.
4. Brush the heated waffle maker with olive oil and add a few tablespoons of the batter. 5. Close the lid and cooking for about 7 minutes depending on your waffle maker.

5. Meanwhile, heat the olive oil in a nonstick pan over medium heat.
6. Season the beef tenderloin with salt and pepper and spread the whole piece of beef tenderloin with Dijon mustard.
7. Cooking on each side for about 4-5 minutes.
8. Serve each chaffle with sour cream and slices of the cooked beef tenderloin.
9. Garnish with freshly chopped spring onion.
10. Serve and enjoy.

Nutrition:

- Calories: 50
- Total Fat: 23 g
- Fiber: 4 g
- Total Carbs: 8 g
- Protein: 2 g

20. Pork Loin Chaffle Sandwich

Preparation time: 10 minutes

Cooking Time: 15 Minutes

Servings: 4

Ingredients:

- 4 eggs
- 1 cup grated Mozzarella cheese
- 1 cup grated parmesan cheese Salt and pepper to taste
- 2 tablespoons cream cheese
- 6 tablespoons coconut flour
- 2 teaspoons baking powder
- Pork loin
- 2 tablespoons olive oil
- 1 pound pork loin
- Salt and pepper to taste
- 2 cloves garlic, minced
- 1 tablespoon freshly chopped thyme
- 2 tablespoons cooking spray to brush the waffle maker
- 4 lettuce leaves for serving
- 4 slices of tomato for serving
- ¼ cup sugar-free mayonnaise for serving

Directions:

1. Preheat the waffle maker.
2. Add the eggs, Mozzarella cheese, parmesan cheese, salt and pepper, cream cheese, coconut flour and baking powder to a bowl.
3. Mix until combined.
4. Brush the heated waffle maker with cooking spray and add a few tablespoons of the batter.

5. Close the lid and cooking for about 7 minutes depending on your waffle maker.
6. Meanwhile, heat the olive oil in a nonstick frying pan and season the pork loin with salt and pepper, minced garlic and freshly chopped thyme.
7. Cooking the pork loin for about 5-minutes on each side.
8. Cut each chaffle in half and add some mayonnaise, lettuce leaf, tomato slice and sliced pork loin on one half.
9. Cover the sandwich with the other chaffle half and serve.

Nutrition:

- Calories: 211
- Fat: 3
- Fiber: 3
- Carbs: 6
- Protein: 8

21. Beef Chaffle Tower

Preparation time: 10 minutes

Cooking Time: 15 Minutes

Servings: 4

Ingredients:

- Batter
- 4 eggs
- 2 cups grated Mozzarella cheese Salt and pepper to taste
- 2 tablespoons almond flour
- 1 teaspoon Italian seasoning
- Beef
- 2 tablespoons butter
- 1 pound beef tenderloin
- Salt and pepper to taste
- 1 teaspoon chili flakes
- Other
- 2 tablespoons cooking spray to brush the waffle maker

Directions:

1. Preheat the waffle maker.
2. Add the eggs, grated Mozzarella cheese, salt and pepper, almond flour and Italian seasoning to a bowl.
3. Mix until everything is fully combined.
4. Brush the heated waffle maker with cooking spray and add a few tablespoons of the batter.
5. Close the lid and cooking for about 7 minutes depending on your waffle maker.
6. Meanwhile, heat the butter in a nonstick frying pan and season the beef tenderloin with salt and pepper and chili flakes.

7. Cooking the beef tenderloin for about 5-minutes on each side.
8. When serving, assemble the chaffle tower by placing one chaffle on a plate, a layer of diced beef tenderloin, another chaffle, another layer of beef, and so on until you finish with the chaffles and beef.
9. Serve and enjoy.

Nutrition:

- Calories: 176
- Total Fat: 3.8 g
- Fiber: 5 g
- Total Carbs: 32.97 g
- Protein: 4 g

22. Red Velvet Chaffle Cake

Preparation Time: 15 minutes

Cooking Time: 28 minutes

Servings: 4

Ingredients

- For the chaffles:
- 2 eggs, beaten
- ½ cup finely grated parmesan cheese
- 2 oz cream cheese, softened
- 2 drops red food coloring
- 1 tsp vanilla extract
- For the frosting:
- 3 tbsp cream cheese, softened
- 1 tbsp sugar-free maple syrup
- ¼ tsp vanilla extract

Directions

1. For the chaffles:
2. Preheat the waffle iron.
3. In a medium bowl, mix all the ingredients for the chaffles.
4. Open the iron and add a quarter of the mixture. Close and cook until crispy, 7 minutes.
5. Transfer the chaffle to a plate and make 3 more chaffles with the remaining batter.
6. For the frosting:

7. In a medium bowl, using a hand mixer, whisk the cream cheese, maple syrup, and vanilla extract until smooth.
8. Assemble the chaffles with the frosting to make the cake.
9. Slice and serve.

Nutrition:

- Calories: 147
- Fats: 9.86 g
- Carbs: 5.22 g
- Net Carbs: 5.22 g
- Protein: 8.57 g

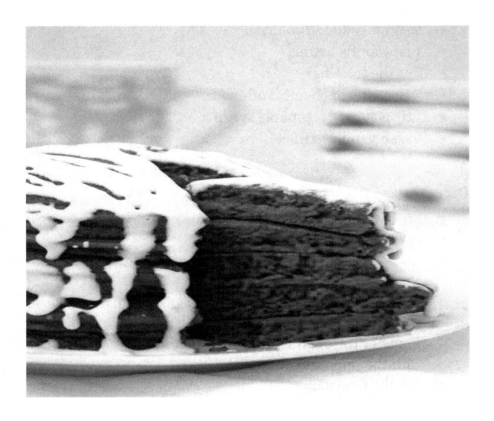

23. Cauliflower-Chaffles And Tomatoes

Preparation Time: 5 minutes

Cooking Time: 15 minutes

Servings: 2

- Ingredients:
- 1/2 cup cauliflower
- 1/4 tsp. garlic powder
- 1/4 tsp. black pepper
- 1/4 tsp. Salt
- 1/2 cup shredded cheddar cheese
- 1 egg
- For Topping
- 1 lettuce leave
- 1 tomato sliced
- 4 oz. cauliflower steamed, mashed
- 1 tsp. sesame seeds

Directions:

1. Add all chaffle ingredients into a blender and mix well.
2. Sprinkle 1/8 shredded cheese on the waffle maker and pour cauliflower mixture in a preheated waffle maker and sprinkle the rest of the cheese over it.
3. Cooking chaffles for about 4-5 minutes until cooked
4. For serving, lay lettuce leaves over chaffle top with steamed cauliflower and tomato.
5. Drizzle sesame seeds on top.
6. Enjoy!

Nutrition:

- Calories: 140
- Total fat: 10 g
- Saturated fat: 5 g
- Sodium: 273 mg
- Phosphorus: 45 mg
- Potassium: 204 mg
- Carbohydrates: 11 g
- Fiber: 6 g
- Protein: 2 g
- Sugar: 2 g

24. Garlic-Chicken Chaffle

Preparation Time: 25 minutes

Cooking Time: 12 minutes

Servings: 2

Ingredients:

- Chicken: 3-4 pieces
- Garlic: 1 clove
- Egg: 1
- Salt
- Lemon juice: ½ tablespoon
- Kewpie mayo: 2 tablespoons
- Mozzarella cheese: ½ cup

Directions:

1. Cooking the chicken in a skillet using salt and a cup of water to boil.
2. With the lid closed, cooking for 18 minutes.
3. Once done, put off the heat and shred the chicken into pieces, then discard all bones.
4. Using another mixing bowl, a mix containing 1/8 cup of cheese, Kewpie mayo, lemon juice and grated garlic. Mix evenly.
5. Preheat and grease the waffle maker. Arrange chaffles on a baking tray with the chicken, then sprinkle cheese on the chaffles.
6. With a closed lid, heat the waffle for 5 minutes until cheese melts and then remove the chaffle.
7. Repeat for the remaining chaffles mixture to make more batter.
8. Serve and warm.

Nutrition:

- Calories: 246
- Total fat: 14 g
- Saturated fat: 6 g
- Sodium: 235 mg
- Phosphorus: 62 mg
- Potassium: 201 mg
- Carbohydrates: 29 g
- Fiber: 3 g
- Protein: 2 g
- Sugar: 13 g

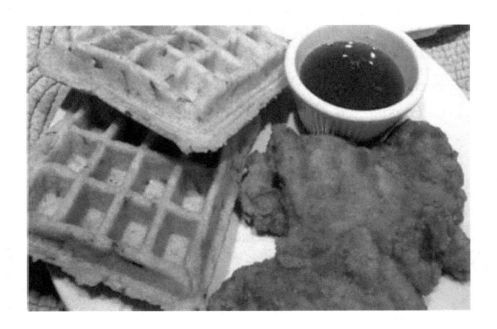

25. Chicken BBQ Chaffle

Preparation time: 32 minutes

Cooking Time: 11 minutes

Servings: 2

Ingredients:

- Chicken: 1/2 cup
- BBQ sauce: 1 tablespoon (sugar-free)
- Egg: 1
- Almond flour: 2 tablespoons
- Cheddar cheese: ½ cup
- Butter: 1 tablespoon

Directions:

1. Melt some butter in a pan with shredded chicken added into it and stir for 11 minutes.
2. Using a mixing bowl, a mixture containing all ingredients with the cooked chicken, then mix evenly.
3. Preheat and grease a waffle maker.
4. Spread the mixture on the base of the waffle maker evenly, and then heat for 7 minutes to a crispy form.
5. Repeat the process for the remaining batter.
6. Serve best hot.

Nutrition:

- Calories: 166
- Total fat: 10 g
- Saturated fat: 1 g
- Sodium: 74 mg
- Phosphorus: 81 mg
- Potassium: 241 mg
- Carbohydrates: 17 g
- Fiber: 4 g
- Protein: 4 g
- Sugar: 2 g

26. Chocolate Cannoli Chaffles

Preparation time: 6 minutes

Cooking Time: 10 Minutes

Servings: 4

Ingredients:

- Cannoli Topping:
- 2 tbsp. granulated swerve
- 4 tbsp. cream cheese
- ¼ tsp. vanilla extract
- ¼ tsp. cinnamon
- 6 tbsp. ricotta cheese
- 1 tsp. lemon juice
- Chaffle:
- 3 tbsp. almond flour
- 1 tbsp. swerve
- 1 egg
- 1/8 tsp. baking powder
- 3/4 tbsp. butter (melted)
- ½ tsp. nutmeg
- 1 tbsp. sugar free chocolate chips
- 1/8 tsp. vanilla extract

Directions:

1. Plug the waffle maker to preheat it and spray it with a non-stick spray.
2. In a mixing bowl, whisk together the egg, butter and vanilla extract.
3. In another mixing bowl, combine the almond flour, baking powder, nutmeg, chocolate chips and swerve.

4. Pour the egg mixture into the flour mixture and mix until the ingredients are well combined and you have formed a smooth batter.
5. Fill your waffle maker with an appropriate amount of the batter and spread out the batter to the edged to cover all the holes on the waffle maker.
6. Close the waffle maker and cooking for about 4 minutes or according to waffle maker's settings.
7. After the baking cycle, remove the chaffle from the waffle maker with a plastic or silicone utensil.
8. Repeat step 5 to 7 until you have cooked all the batter into waffles.
9. For the topping, pour the cream cheese into a blender and add the ricotta, lemon juice, cinnamon, vanilla and swerve sweetener. Blend until smooth and fluffy.
10. Spread the cream over the chaffles and enjoy.

Nutrition:

- Total calories: 102
- Protein: 13 g
- Carbs: 4 g
- Fat: 4 g
- Fiber: 0 g

27. Broccoli and Cheese Chaffle

Preparation time: 5 minutes

Cooking Time: 15 Minutes

Servings: 1

Ingredients:

1/3 cup broccoli (finely chopped) ½ tsp. oregano

1/8 tsp. salt or to taste

1/8 tsp. ground black pepper or to taste' ½ tsp. garlic powder

- ½ tsp. onion powder
- 1 egg (beaten)
- 4 tbsp. shredded cheddar cheese

Directions:

1. Plug the waffle maker to preheat it and spray it with a non-stick cooking spray.
2. In a mixing bowl, combine the cheese, oregano, pepper, garlic, salt and onion. Add the egg and mix until the ingredients are well combined.
3. Fold in the chopped broccoli.
4. Pour an appropriate amount of the batter into your waffle maker and spread out the batter to the edges to cover all the holes on the waffle maker.
5. Close the waffle maker and cooking for about 6-8 until the chaffle is browned. Cooking time may vary in some waffle makers.
6. After the cooking cycle, use a silicone or plastic utensil to remove the chaffle from the waffle maker.
7. Repeat step 4 to 6 until you have cooked all the batter into chaffles.
8. Serve and top with sour cream as desired.

Nutrition:

- Total calories: 331
- Protein: 19 g
- Carbs: 6 g
- Fat: 26 g
- Fiber: 0 g

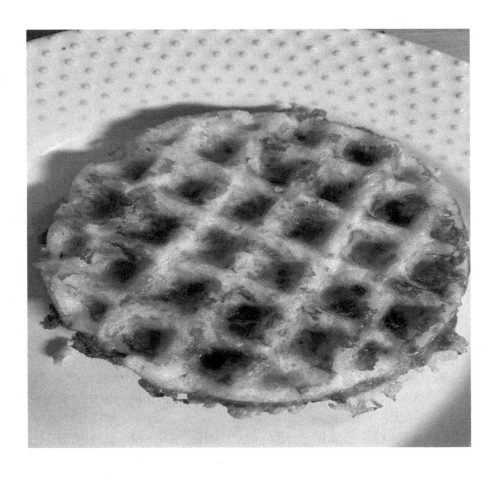

28. Eggnog Chaffle

Preparation time: 5 minutes

Cooking Time: 5 Minutes

Servings: 2

Ingredients:

- 2 tbsp. coconut flour
- ½ tsp. baking powder
- 1 tsp. cinnamon
- 2 tbsp. cream cheese
- 2 tsp. swerve
- 1/8 tsp. salt
- 1/8 tsp. nutmeg
- 1 egg (beaten)
- 4 tbsp. keto eggnog
- Eggnog Filling:
- 4 tbsp. keto eggnog
- ¼ tsp. vanilla extract
- ¼ cup heavy cream
- 2 tsp. granulated swerve
- 1/8 tsp. nutmeg

Directions:

1. Plug the waffle maker to preheat it and spray it with a non-stick cooking spray.
2. Combine the coconut flour, baking powder, swerve, salt, cinnamon and nutmeg in a mixing bowl.
3. In another mixing bowl, whisk together the eggnog, cream cheese and egg.
4. Pour in the egg mixture into the flour mixture and mix until the ingredients are well combined.

5. Fill the waffle maker with an appropriate amount of the batter. Spread out the batter to cover all the holes on the waffle maker.
6. Close the waffle maker and cooking for about 5 minutes or according to your waffle maker's settings.
7. After the baking cycle, remove the chaffle from the waffle maker with a plastic or silicone utensil.
8. Repeat step 5 to 7 until you have cooked all the batter into chaffles.
9. For the eggnog cream, whisk together the cream cheese, heavy cream, vanilla and eggnog. Add the swerve and nutmeg; mix until the ingredients are well combined.
10. Top the chaffles with the eggnog cream and enjoy

Nutrition:

- Total calories: 325
- Protein: 40 g
- Carbs: 6 g
- Fat: 16 g
- Fiber: 0 g

29. Double Cheese Chaffles Plus Mayonnaise Dip

Preparation time: 5 minutes

Cooking Time: 8 Minutes

Servings: 2

Ingredients:

- Chaffles
- ½ cup Mozzarella cheese, shredded
- 1 tablespoon Parmesan cheese, shredded
- 1 organic egg
- ¾ teaspoon coconut flour
- ¼ teaspoon organic baking powder
- 1/8 teaspoon Italian seasoning
- Pinch of salt
- Dip
- ¼ cup mayonnaise
- Pinch of garlic powder
- Pinch of ground black pepper

Directions:

1. Preheat a mini waffle iron and then grease it.
2. For chaffles: In a medium bowl, put all ingredients and with a fork, mix until well combined. Place half of the mixture into preheated waffle iron and cooking for about 3-4 minutes.
3. Repeat with the remaining mixture.
4. Meanwhile, for dip: in a bowl, mix together the cream and stevia.
5. Serve warm chaffles alongside the dip.

Nutrition:

- Total calories: 408
- Protein: 33 g
- Carbs: 21 g
- Fat: 22 g
- Fiber: 2.8 g

30. Yellow Sweet Cake Chaffle

Preparation time: 5 minutes

Cooking Time: 18 Minutes

Servings: 10

Ingredients:

- 1 tbsp. toasted pecans (chopped)
- 2 tbsp. granulated swerve
- 1 tsp. pumpkin spice
- 1 tsp. baking powder
- ½ shredded carrots
- 2 tbsp. butter (melted)
- 1 tsp. cinnamon
- 1 tsp. vanilla extract (optional)
- 2 tbsp. heavy whipping cream ¾ cup almond flour
- 1 egg (beaten)
- Butter cream cheese frosting:
- ½ cup cream cheese (softened)
- ¼ cup butter (softened)
- ½ tsp. vanilla extract
- ¼ cup granulated swerve

Directions:

1. Plug the chaffle maker to preheat it and spray it with a non-stick cooking spray.
2. In a mixing bowl, combine the almond flour, cinnamon, carrot, pumpkin spice and swerve.
3. In another mixing bowl, whisk together the eggs, butter, heavy whipping cream and vanilla extract.
4. Pour the flour mixture into the egg mixture and mix until you form a smooth batter.

5. Fold in the chopped pecans.
6. Pour in an appropriate amount of the batter into your waffle maker and spread out the batter to the edges to cover all the holes on the waffle maker.
7. Close the waffle maker and cooking for about 3 minutes or according to your waffle maker's settings.
8. After the cooking cycle, use a plastic or silicone utensil to remove the chaffle from the waffle maker.
9. Repeat step 6 to 8 until you have cooked all the batter into chaffles.
10. For the frosting, combine the cream cheese and cutter int a mixer and mix until well combined.
11. Add the swerve and vanilla extract and slowly until the sweetener is well incorporated. Mix on high
12. until the frosting is fluffy.
13. Place one chaffle on a flat surface and spread some cream frosting over it. Layer another chaffle over the first one a spread some cream over it too.
14. Repeat step 12 until you have assembled all the chaffles into a cake.
15. Cut and serve.

Nutrition:

- Total calories: 275
- Protein: 26 g
- Carbs: 12 g
- Fat: 15 g
- Fiber: 3.5 g

31. Bacon Jalapeno Popper Chaffle

Preparation time: 5 minutes

Cooking Time: 10 Minutes

Servings: 3

Ingredients:

- 4 slices bacon (diced)
- 3 eggs
- 3 tbsp. coconut flour
- 1 tsp. baking powder
- ¼ tsp. salt
- ½ tsp. oregano
- A pinch of onion powder
- A pinch of garlic powder
- ½ cup cream cheese
- 1 cup shredded cheddar cheese
- 2 jalapeno pepper (deseeded and chopped)
- ½ cup sour cream

Directions:

1. Plug the waffle maker to preheat it and spray it with a non-stick cooking spray.
2. Heat up a frying pan over medium to high heat. Add the bacon and sauté until the bacon is brown and crispy.
3. Use a slotted spoon to transfer the bacon to a paper towel lined plate to drain.
4. In a mixing bowl, combine the coconut flour, baking powder, salt, oregano, onion and garlic.
5. In another mixing bowl, whisk together the egg and cream cheese until well combined.

6. Add the cheddar cheese and mix. Pour in the flour mixture and mix until you form a smooth batter.

7. Pour an appropriate amount of the batter into the waffle maker and spread the batter to the edges to cover all the holes on the waffle maker.

8. Close the waffle maker and cooking for about 5 minutes or according to waffle maker's settings.

9. After the cooking cycle, use a plastic or silicone utensil to remove the chaffle from the waffle maker.

10. Repeat step 7 to 9 until you have cooked all the batter into chaffles.

11. Serve warm and top with sour cream, crispy bacon and jalapeno slices.

Nutrition:

- Total calories: 351
- Protein: 17 g
- Carbs: 6 g
- Fat: 27 g
- Fiber: 1.6 g

32. Apple Pie Chaffle

Preparation time: 5 minutes

Cooking Time: 6 Minutes

Servings: 2

Ingredients:

- 1 egg (beaten)
- 1 tbsp. almond flour
- 1 big apple (finely chopped)
- 1 tbsp. heavy whipping cream
- 1 tsp. cinnamon
- 1 tbsp. granulated swerve
- ½ tsp. vanilla extract
- 1/3 cup Mozzarella cheese
- Topping:
- ¼ tbsp. sugar free maple syrup

Directions:

1. Plug the waffle maker and preheat it. Spray it with non-stick spray.
2. In a large mixing bowl, combine the swerve, almond flour, mozzarella, cinnamon and chopped apple.
3. Add the eggs, vanilla extract and heavy whipping cream. Mix until all the ingredients are well combined.
4. Fill the waffle maker with the batter and spread out the batter to the edges of the waffle maker to all the holes on it.
5. Close the lid of the waffle maker and cooking for about 4 minute or according to waffle maker's settings.
6. After the cooking cycle, remove the chaffle from the waffle maker with a plastic or silicone utensil.

7. Repeat step 4 to 6 until you have cooked all the batter into chaffles.
8. Serve and top with maple syrup.

Nutrition:

- Total calories: 347
- Protein: 25 g
- Carbs: 3 g
- Fat: 24 g
- Fiber: 0 g

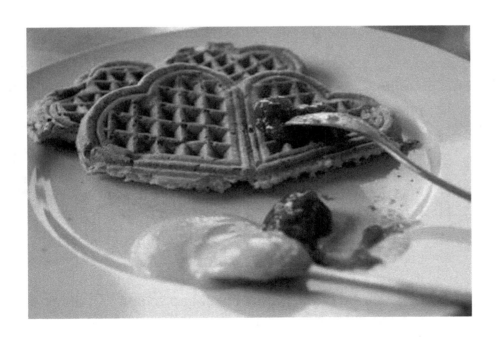

33. French Toast Chaffle Sticks

Preparation time: 5 minutes

Cooking Time: 40 Minutes

Servings: 8

Ingredients:

- 6 organic eggs
- 2 cups Mozzarella cheese, shredded ¼ cup coconut flour
- 2 tablespoons powdered erythritol
- 1 teaspoon ground cinnamon
- 1 tablespoon butter, melted

Directions:

1. Preheat your oven to 350°F and line a large baking sheet with a greased piece of foil.
2. Preheat a waffle iron and then grease it.
3. In a bowl, add 4 eggs and beat well.
4. Add the cheese, coconut flour, erythritol and ½ teaspoon of cinnamon and mix until well combined.
5. Place ¼ of the mixture into preheated waffle iron and cooking for about 6-8 minutes.
6. Repeat with the remaining mixture.
7. Set the chaffles aside to cool.
8. Cut each chaffle into 4 strips.
9. In a large bowl, add the remaining eggs and cinnamon and beat until well combined.
10. Dip the chaffle sticks in the egg mixture evenly.
11. Arrange the chaffle sticks onto the prepared baking sheet in a single layer.
12. Bake for about 10 minutes.
13. Remove the baking sheet from oven and brush the top of each stick with the melted butter.

14. Flip the stick and bake for about 6-8 minutes.
15. Serve immediately.

Nutrition:

- Total Calories: 96
- Protein: 7 g
- Carbs: 11 g
- Fat: 5 g
- Fiber: 2.3 g

34. Sweet Brownie Chaffle

Preparation time: 5 minutes

Cooking Time: 14 Minutes

Servings: 2

Ingredients:

- 1 large egg
- ¼ tsp. baking powder
- ½ tsp. vanilla extract
- ½ tsp. ginger
- 2 tbsp. cream cheese (melted)
- 1 ½ tsp. cocoa powder
- 1 tbsp. swerve
- Topping:
- ½ tsp. vanilla extract.
- ½ tsp. cinnamon
- ¼ tsp. liquid stevia
- 2 tbsp. heavy cream
- 6 tbsp. cream cheese (melted)

Directions:

1. Plug the waffle maker to preheat it and spray it with a non-stick cooking spray.
2. In a mixing bowl, combine the swerve, cocoa powder, ginger and baking powder.
3. In another mixing bowl, whisk together the cream cheese, egg and vanilla.
4. Pour the cocoa powder mixture into the egg mixture and mix until the ingredients are well combined.

5. Fill the waffle maker with an appropriate amount of batter and spread the batter to the edges to cover all the holes on the waffle maker.
6. Close the waffle maker and cooking for about 7 minutes or according to your waffle maker's settings.
7. After the cooking cycle, use a silicone or plastic utensil to remove the chaffle from the waffle maker. Set aside to cool completely
8. Repeat step 5 to 7 until all the batter has been cooked into chaffles.
9. For the filling, combine the vanilla, cream cheese, stevia, cinnamon and heavy cream in a mixing bowl. Mix until well combined.
10. Spread the cream frosting over the surface of one chaffle and cover with another chaffle.
11. Place the filled chaffles in a refrigerator and chill for about 15 minutes.
12. Serve and enjoy.

Nutrition:

- Total Calories: 165
- Protein: 3 g
- Carbs: 15 g
- Fat: 13 g
- Fiber: 3.7 g

SPECIAL CHAFFLE RECIPES

35. Banana Cheddar Chaffle

Preparation Time: 5 minutes

Cooking Time: 10 minutes

Servings: 4

Ingredients:

- Egg: 1
- Cream cheese: 1 tbsp.
- Cheddar cheese: ½ cup
- Banana extract: ¼ tbsp.
- Vanilla extract: ½ tsp.
- Monkfruit sweetener: 1 tbsp.
- Caramel sauce: 2 tbsp. (sugar-free)

Directions:

1. Preheat a mini waffle maker if needed and grease it
2. In a mixing bowl, beat eggs and add all the chaffle ingredients except caramel sauce
3. Mix them all well
4. Pour the mixture to the lower plate of the waffle maker and spread it evenly to cover the plate properly
5. Close the lid
6. Cooking for at least 4 minutes to get the desired crunch
7. Remove the chaffle from the heat and keep aside for around one minute
8. Make as many chaffles as your mixture and waffle maker allow
9. Serve with caramel sauce

Nutrition:

- Calories: 233
- Fat: 12 g
- Fiber: 6 g
- Carbs: 25 g
- Protein: 23 g

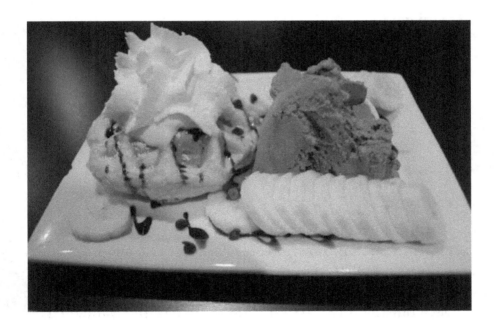

36. Cantaloupe Chaffles

Preparation Time: 5 minutes

Cooking Time: 17 minutes

Servings: 4

Ingredients:

- Eggs: 2
- Cheddar cheese: 1 cup shredded
- Cantaloupe: 1 cup mashed
- Coconut flour: 2 tsp.
- Vanilla: ½ tsp.

Directions:

1. Preheat your mini waffle iron if needed and grease it
2. Mix all the ingredients in a bowl and whisk
3. Cooking your mixture in the mini waffle iron for at least 4 minutes
4. Make as many chaffles as your mixture and waffle maker allow

Nutrition:

- Calories: 98
- Fat: 21 g
- Fiber: 10 g
- Carbs: 20 g
- Protein: 19 g

37. Creamy Pistachios Chaffles

Preparation Time: 5 minutes

Cooking Time: 10 minutes

Servings: 2

Ingredients:

- Egg: 1
- Mozzarella cheese: ½ cup shredded
- Swerve/Monkfruit: 1 tsp.
- Vanilla extract: 1/2 tsp.
- Coconut flour: 1 tbsp.
- Cream: ¼ cup
- Pistachios: ½ cup chopped

Directions:

1. Add all the chaffle ingredients in a bowl and whisk
2. Preheat your mini waffle iron if needed and grease it
3. Cooking your mixture in the mini waffle iron for at least 4 minutes
4. Make as many chaffles as you can and spread cream or low-carb ice cream on top

Nutrition:

- Calories: 220
- Fat: 8 g
- Fiber: 10 g
- Carbs: 36 g
- Protein: 10 g

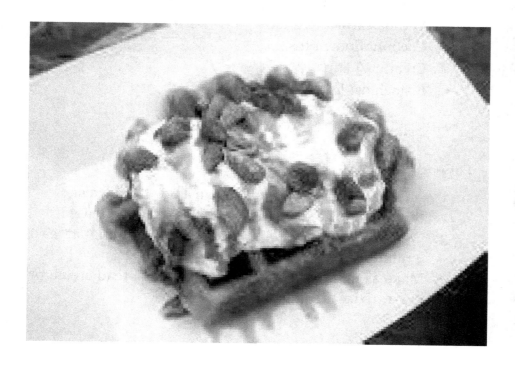

38. Chocolate Keto Chaffle

Preparation Time: 5 minutes

Cooking Time: 10 minutes

Servings: 2

Ingredients:

- Egg: 3
- Butter: ½ cup
- Chocolate chips: ½ cup (sugar-free)
- Truvia: ¼ cup (you can use any other sweetener as well)
- Vanilla extract: 1 tsp.

Directions:

1. In a bowl, add butter and chocolate chips and microwave for one minute only
2. Remove from microwave and stir to melt the chocolate using the butter's heat and set aside
3. Preheat a mini waffle maker if needed and grease it
4. In a mixing bowl, beat eggs, and add truvia and vanilla and blend to froth
5. Now add chocolate and butter in the mixture
6. Mix them all well and pour the mixture to the lower plate of the waffle maker
7. Close the lid
8. Cooking for at least 5 minutes to get the desired crunch
9. Remove the chaffle from the heat
10. Make as many chaffles as your mixture and waffle maker allow
11. Serve with your favorite toppings and enjoy!

Nutrition:

- Calories: 188
- Fat: 9 g
- Fiber: 6 g
- Carbs: 20 g
- Protein: 45 g

39. Fresh Strawberries Chaffle

Preparation Time: 5 minutes

Cooking Time: 10 minutes

Servings: 2

Ingredients:

- Egg: 1
- Mozzarella cheese: ½ cup
- Almond flour: 1 tbsp.
- Swerve: 1½ tbsp.
- Vanilla extract: ¼ tsp.
- Whipped cream: 2 tbsp.
- Strawberry: 4

Directions:

1. Preheat a mini waffle maker if needed
2. Chop fresh strawberries and mix with half tablespoon of granulated swerve and keep it aside
3. In a mixing bowl, beat eggs and add Mozzarella cheese, almond flour, granulated swerve, and vanilla extract
4. Mix them all well and pour the mixture to the lower plate of the waffle maker
5. Close the lid
6. Cooking for at least 4 minutes to get the desired crunch
7. Remove the chaffle from the heat and keep aside for around two minutes
8. Make as many chaffles as your mixture and waffle maker allow
9. Serve with the fresh strawberries mixture you made with the whipped cream on top

Nutrition:

- Calories: 220
- Fat: 25 g
- Fiber: 16 g
- Carbs: 15 g
- Protein: 35 g

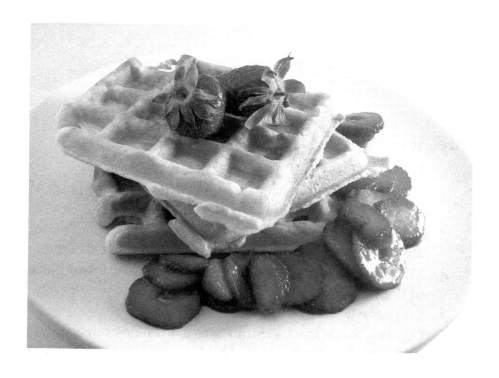

40. Cinnamon Peach Chaffles

Preparation Time: 5 minutes

Cooking Time: 20 minutes

Servings: 4

Ingredients:

- Cheddar cheese: 1/3 cup
- Egg: 1
- Peach puree: ¼ cup
- Monkfruit sweetener: 1 tsp.
- Cinnamon powder: 2 tbsp.
- Baking powder: 1/4 teaspoon
- Mozzarella cheese: 1/3 cup

Directions:

1. Mix cheddar cheese, egg, peach puree, monkfruit sweetener, and baking powder together in a bowl
2. Preheat your waffle iron and grease it
3. In your mini waffle iron, shred half of the Mozzarella cheese
4. Add the mixture to your mini waffle iron
5. Again, shred the remaining Mozzarella cheese on the mixture
6. Cooking till the desired crisp is achieved
7. Make as many chaffles as your mixture and waffle maker allow
8. Sprinkle cinnamon on top before serving

Nutrition:

- Calories: 178
- Fat: 7 g
- Fiber: 6 g
- Carbs: 12 g
- Protein: 25 g

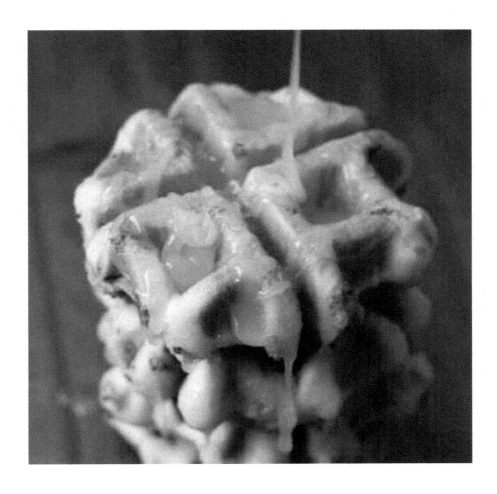

CONCLUSION

C haffles is the amazing new invention you've been waiting for. It's a revolutionary, patent-pending, and 100% vegan protein bar with a thousand uses.

What are chaffles? Chaffles is a delicious new product that can be used to replace the high fat and high sugar snacks in your diet like cheese chips or chocolate bars. It's also gluten-free, vegan, non-GMO, low in sodium and preservative free! The best part is that chaffles taste just as good as candy! You'll never want anything else again after trying this life changing snack.

The combination of protein and savory chaffle taste will keep you wanting to eat more every time. Chaffles are also a great substitute for those times that you feel like having something sweet, but want something healthy with a lot of flavor.

Chaffles come in an assortment of flavors like Pecan Pie or Cherry Pie and can be served with a drizzle of your favorite nut butter or cinnamon sugar for an awesome snack. Or you can create your own combinations by mixing them up the way that makes your mouth water.

Chaffles are great for both kids and adults. They're the perfect snack to bring on a hike for an afternoon treat or to eat on a road trip or flights. Even better, they create a new way for parents to get their kids to eat protein without them even knowing what they're eating. Now if you want your children to enjoy healthy food without complaining, chaffles will be your best friend.

No matter what you eat chaffles with, it will never disappoint! Have it with chicken noodle soup or mashed potatoes for dinner or have it with salad at lunch.

Chaffle is a perfect combination for keto dieters. Besides, keto diet is always low in carbs and high in fat so chaffle is an amazing option for it.

Chaffles are very versatile and can be used as a spread for your favorite bagel or toast, or even on top of a pizza before baking it. You can also use chaffles as an ingredient for your own meals like pancakes, pies, donuts, breads and so much more!

Chaffle comes in two different flavors: savory and sweet. The savory flavor is more of a BBQ flavor while the sweet flavor is more cookie dough style. The savory chaffles are perfect for replacing things like bread and crackers, while sweet chaffles can be used as a dessert or drink! You can also add chaffle to your favorite dessert recipes for an amazing taste.

Chaffles are the most unique tasting protein bar around that is also good for you. You won't believe how good they taste until you try them for yourself. This incredible product is sure to revolutionize your snacking experience and change the way you think about eating healthy forever.

Always remember when making your own chaffle recipes, you can choose from almost any combination of things like fruits, cereals, nuts and seeds. You can even use different types of chocolate in some recipes. Anything goes with chaffle!

What's even more exciting is that chaffles come in many sizes to fit anyone's taste and diet.

It's time to ditch your unhealthy snacks for life changing chaffles!

CPSIA information can be obtained
at www.ICGtesting.com
Printed in the USA
BVHW041747220621
610214BV00012B/2430